Is It Safe to Go to the Dental Office?

Yes. This book describes the many measures, the behind-the-scenes activities, that the dentist and staff undertake to ensure that you are not exposed to disease-causing microbes (germs) in the dental office. These measures have been developed over the years in response to concern about the possibility of transmitting or contracting diseases, particularly hepatitis and HIV, in various health-care settings. The measures are many, and vary from the simple—such as hand washing or the disinfection of a countertop—to the elaborate, such as the sterilization of instruments with high-pressure steam.

Be assured that your dental office has never been safer.

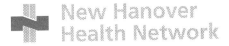

Why Is the Dental Team Concerned About Infection Control?

Members of the dental team care very much about your well-being and health. Dental-care providers abide by a code of ethics established by the American Dental Association. This code of ethics has, as its primary goal, your safety. Dating back to Hippocrates, this imperative of health-care providers declares, "Do no harm." Abiding by these ethics helps guarantee quality care while minimizing any associated risks.

Infection-control procedures are one way of caring for both you and the dental team by minimizing the risk of transmission of *pathogens* (disease-causing microbes, or germs) from dental-care provider to patient and patient to dental-care provider.

The dental team puts forth considerable effort in preparing the dental operatory for individual patients; most of this preparation is accomplished long before you are seated in the dental chair.

Dentistry's Leadership in Infection Control

In health care, dentistry has been at the forefront of the development of new products and procedures that reduce the potential for disease transmission in the office setting. Recently, new dental sterilizers that process instruments faster and more effectively have been introduced. Likewise, protective equipment routinely used by dentists, such as certain types of masks and face shields, is now being used by those in other medical specialties.

Studies have shown that dentists are in fact more willing and accommodating in practicing infection-control techniques than other health-care providers.

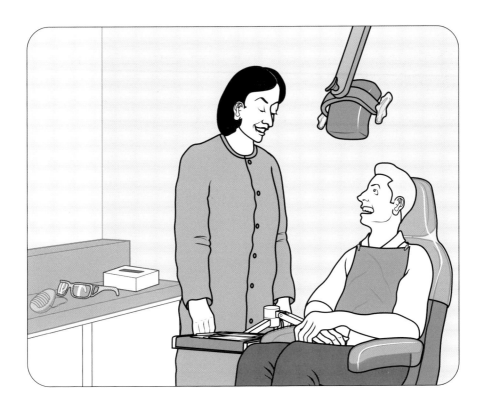

How Are Infectious Diseases Transmitted?

Infectious diseases can be transmitted in several ways, including direct contact with contaminated fluids (such as blood or saliva); indirect contact with contaminated dental instruments or other dental equipment; and contact with air-borne pathogens. However, infections need four conditions to occur:

1. The person exposed to the infectious microbe must be *susceptible*. A variety of factors influence susceptibility, including general state of health, and previous infections or immunizations, which sometimes result in the creation of protective *antibodies*. For instance, individuals successfully immunized against the hepatitis B virus are no longer susceptible to infection by this virus.

2. A specific number of infectious pathogens must be present. The body's immune system can usually resist a limited number of microbes, but if the microbes become too numerous, they overwhelm the body's defenses and cause an infection.

3. The microbes must be highly infectious. Weakened viruses can actually be put to use; many vaccines consist of weakened viruses that do not *cause disease* but instead enable the body to form protective proteins—antibodies—that make individuals immune to disease.

4. Pathogens must enter the body in an appropriate manner. Depending on the microbe and where it enters the body, infection may or may not occur. For instance, if HIV enters the mouth, infection will most probably not occur. But if it enters the blood stream directly, an infection will probably occur.

Infection-control procedures are designed to disrupt these four conditions, reducing the possibility of disease transmission dramatically.

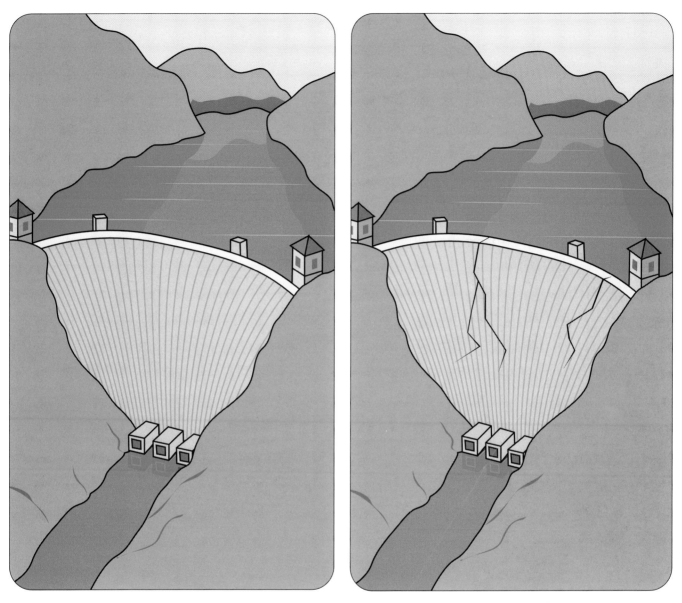

When germs become too numerous, they overwhelm the body's defenses, like water breaking through a dam.

What Exactly Is Infection Control?

Infection control is a way to minimize the transmission of microbes in the dental office. Potentially, diseases could be transmitted in a dental setting in three ways—from patient to dental-care provider, from patient to patient, and from dental-care provider to patient.

Infection-control procedures *arrest* disease transmission by using different methods—such as physical barriers, chemical agents, and heat.

Universal Precautions

Because the dental team cannot identify all patients who harbor disease-causing microbes, a system called *universal precautions* is used. Universal precautions simply means that *all* patients are treated with the *same* type of precautions. It assures that even if a patient does not know that he or she is infectious, protection for the dental team and other patients is assured. Universal precautions dramatically reduces the spread of potential harmful diseases in the dental setting.

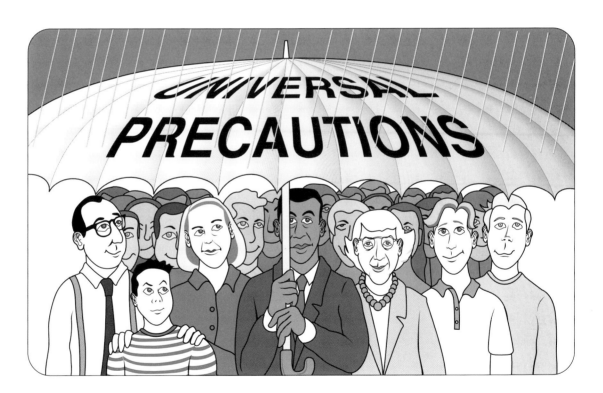

Everyone Benefits from Infection Control

Many people don't know that the dental-care providers are at higher risk of contracting infectious diseases from their patients than are patients from dental-care providers. However, since the introduction of universal precautions and recommendations for vaccination against pathogens such as the hepatitis B virus, the rate of infectious diseases acquired by health-care providers has decreased dramatically.

Federal and state governments have laws and regulations that require employers to provide safe workplace conditions for every employee. These laws and regulations require employers to provide employees with appropriate protection against infection. These infection-control procedures benefit both you and members of the dental team.

Who Sets Infection Control Guidelines?

Numerous federal regulations from the Centers for Disease Control and Prevention (CDC) and Occupational Safety and Health Administration (OSHA) advise health-care professionals, like dentists, how to implement appropriate infection control measures. State and local guidelines are also usually based on the recommendations of CDC and OSHA. Failure to follow these guidelines can result in legal action against the dental office.

Professional organizations, such as the American Dental Association (ADA), issue infection-control guidelines for dentists. These recommendations are revised and updated continually by world leaders in the field of infection control.

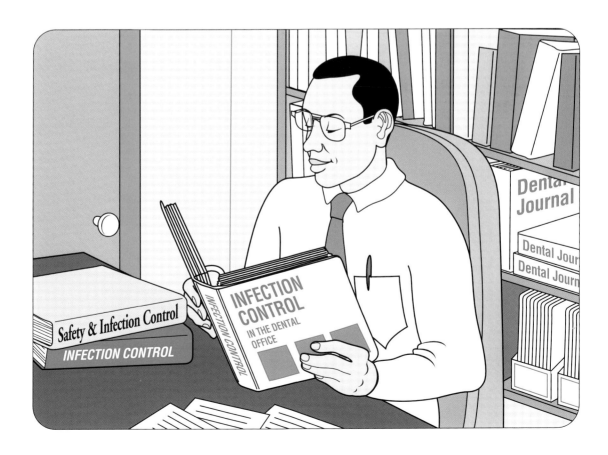

How Is Infection Control Implemented?

Approaches to infection control may vary among dental offices, but the same basic principles underlie them. All dental team members are offered regular training programs, free hepatitis B virus vaccinations, and frequent updates on the latest techniques and principles in infection control. Governing the day-to-day implementation of infection control is the use of *universal precautions*—treating every patient as if he or she were a carrier of an infectious disease. It is achieved in several ways:

1. Using physical barriers for protection. In the dental office, you might see chair covers or other protective devices, such as masks, gloves, eye wear, or disposable gowns. These physical barriers are for your benefit, as well as for the protection of the dental team. These barriers are changed between patients.

2. Using disposable items. In addition to the disposable physical barriers, dentists use, as much as possible, disposable bibs, disposable cups, and disposable saliva ejectors (suction tips). Such items help minimize the spread of infection.

3. Cleaning instruments and equipment thoroughly between patients. This involves destroying or reducing the number of microbes that have contaminated dental equipment that is not disposable. The dental team also takes extra care to practice clean work methods.

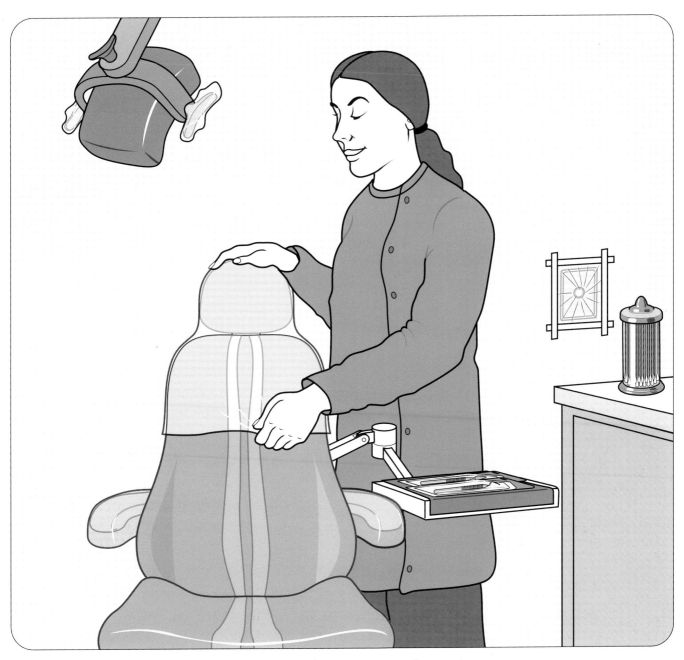

A dentist prepares the treatment area for a patient.

4. Attempting to identify as many patients as possible who are infectious. This also enables the referral of patients for appropriate medical care. Furthermore, certain infectious conditions may warrant a change of dental procedures.

The dentist conducts a review of your medical forms and performs an oral examination. You can help by filling out your medical history form as honestly and completely as possible. The dentist, or another member of the dental team, can help those who have problems understanding or filling out the form. All information on the form is confidential, and no one in the dental office can disclose information without your consent.

Because many people see their dentist more frequently than their physician, dentists are in a good position (and even feel obligated) to identify possible medical conditions. Helping you identify any such conditions is the first step toward ensuring that you are getting the care you need.

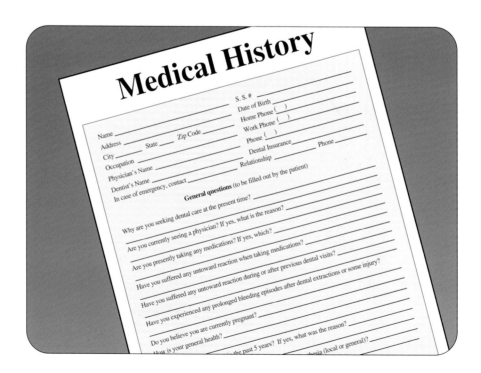

What Are the Infection-Control Procedures?

The prevention of contamination or transmission can be described by two simple concepts: *barriers* to micro-organisms and *eliminators* of micro-organisms.

Asepsis

Asepsis is the first way to prevent contamination. In asepsis, microbes are not necessarily destroyed, but their ability to infect is interrupted. In dentistry, asepsis is achieved in two ways.

1. Hand washing. The dental team washes their hands before and after every patient.
2. Barriers and coverings. Physical barriers, such as gloves, gowns, masks, and disposable coverings placed on items such as switches and controls, prevent the possibility of contamination.

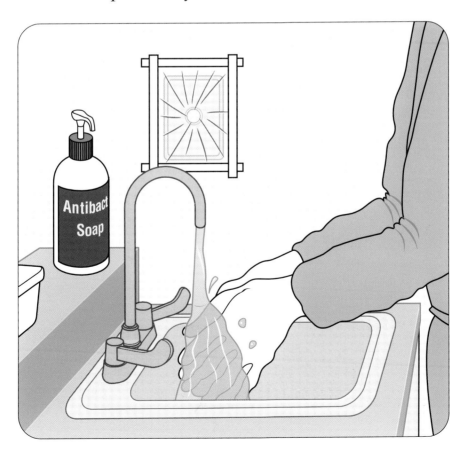

Why Does the Dental Team Wear . . . ?

You may notice the dental staff wearing masks, gloves, gowns, and protective eye wear. These *barrier* methods of infection control do not destroy disease-causing microbes but prevent contaminating sources from infecting the dental staff and patients. These protective garbs may be changed and/or discarded, or disinfected, between patients.

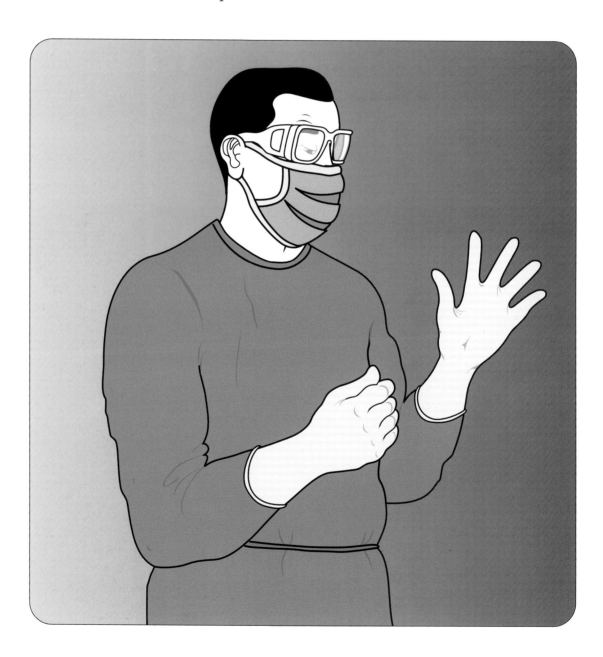

Gloves

Gloves are worn to prevent exposing the dental-care provider's skin to the microbes in blood, saliva, or mucous membranes. Gloves are changed between patients, and dental team members wash their hands, both before putting on their gloves and after removing them. Some prefer to wear sterile gloves or surgical gloves for certain procedures, as well as regular vinyl gloves. Latex gloves, known as examination gloves, are appropriate for all general dental procedures and are most commonly used.

Infection control guidelines even address the way gloves are put on, taken off, and disposed of.

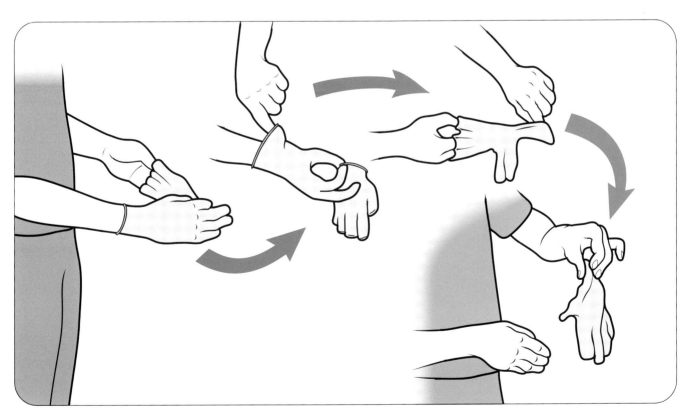

Even seemingly simple procedures are standardized for safety. Health-care providers remove gloves in a particular way to avoid contact with potentially contaminated surfaces.

Masks

Properly fitting masks are worn to protect the dental team member's face from exposure to blood or saliva that may be splattered from the patient's mouth during the course of a normal dental visit. *Dental aerosol* is generated during drilling of teeth and during cleaning of teeth with a cavitron. The highest concentration of micro-organisms from dental aerosol is found within a two-foot radius of the patient. Any team member within this radius should wear a mask.

Masks also protect the patient from exposure to upper respiratory–tract pathogens that a member of the dental team may be harboring.

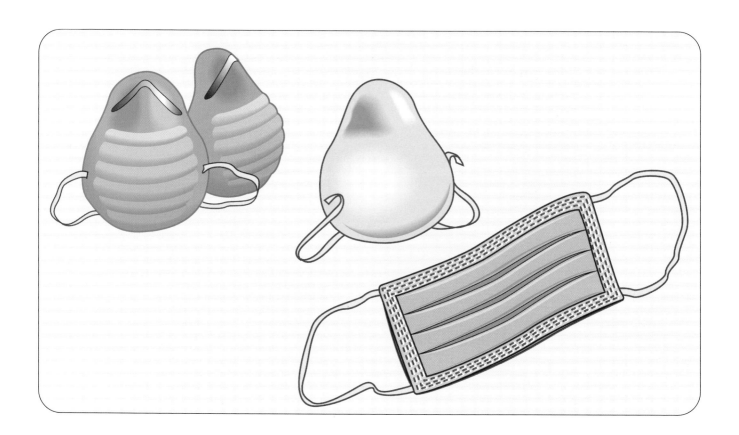

Glasses

Protective eye wear, in the form of glasses with side shields or a face shield, is used to protect the eyes from blood, saliva splatters, and dental aerosol. In some dental offices, patients are also asked to wear protective eye wear to minimize the chance of physical injury to their eyes during certain dental procedures.

Gowns

Members of the dental team wear gowns during procedures that generate dental aerosol. These gowns are usually fluid-resistant and act as a physical barrier to prevent exposure from aerosols and other matter to street clothes and bare skin. These gowns can be changed between patients or when visibly soiled. Many dental offices employ outside contractors to clean and prepare nondisposable gowns before they are used with patients.

What Is Disinfection?

Disinfection is a process whereby most of the organisms that cause disease are killed by chemical agents. Disinfection is distinguished from sterilization, a more complete method of killing microbes. Large objects that can't be sterilized—such as countertops and dental chairs—are disinfected between patients, as are certain plastic or rubber instruments that would be destroyed under the conditions required for sterilization.

Many types of disinfectants are available, but dentists usually choose products registered with the Environmental Protection Agency (EPA) and approved by the American Dental Association (ADA). All disinfectants used in dental offices are designed to destroy even very resistant bacteria, such as *M. tuberculosis*. Premixed disinfection solutions are changed on a regular basis, as determined by their expiration date, to assure maximum effectiveness.

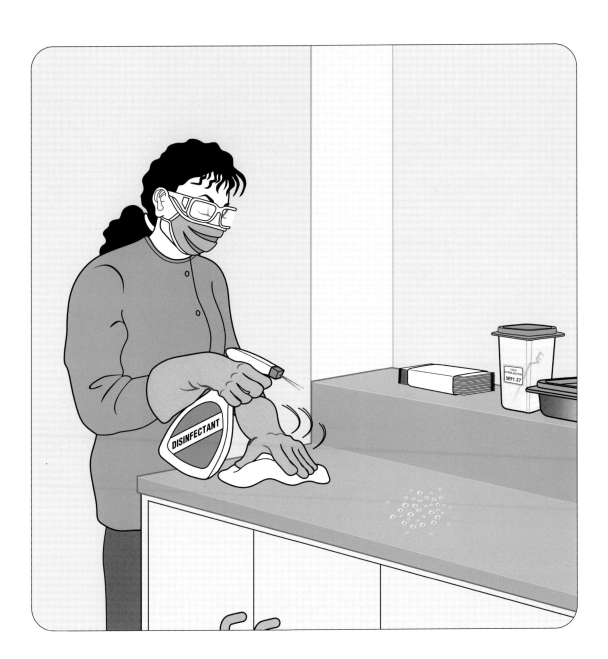

What Is Sterilization?

Sterilization is the ultimate process to *destroy* all living micro-organisms, including *spores* (reproductive bodies) of the hardiest bacteria and fungi. This process is facilitated by initial removal of material by cleaning and the use of an ultrasonic device.

An item can be sterilized in a number of ways. Commonly, instruments are treated with high-pressure steam for an extended period of time. This process is known as *autoclaving*.

Autoclaving process

In *autoclaving*, instruments (which are first cleaned, dried, and placed in a special steam-penetrable wrap), are subjected to pressurized steam for 15 to 20 minutes. The machine that performs this process is called an *autoclave*. After autoclaving, the instruments are left in their protective packaging until they are ready to be used in the treatment of a patient.

Chemiclaving process

Another acceptable method of sterilizing instruments is *chemiclaving*, or subjecting the instruments to heated and pressurized chemical solutions. This method is similar to autoclaving but requires a higher temperature and pressure and is therefore not suited for all types of dental instruments.

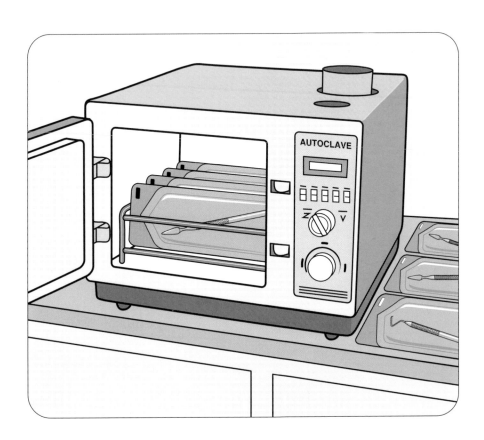

Dry heat process

The dry heat process is another way of sterilizing dental instruments. This method requires even greater heat. New sterilizers with shorter heating cycles using this method have been popular for the sterilization of special instruments such as orthodontic tools.

Cold sterilization

For items that would be damaged by the high heat involved in other sterilization processes, a nonheated liquid sterilization procedure is used. This involves soaking the contaminated object in a chemical solution, such as glutaraldehyde, for about 10 hours.

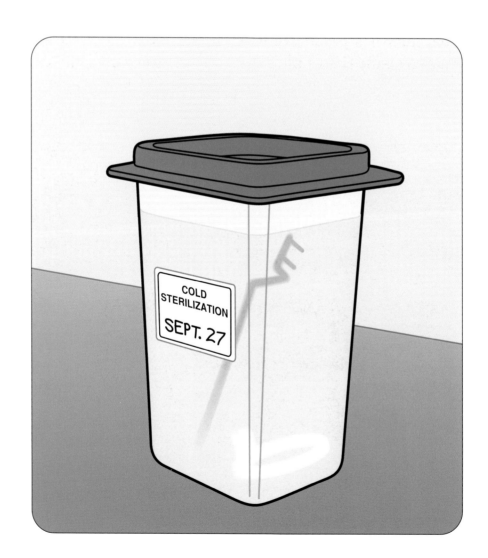

Do All Dental Instruments Need to Be Sterilized?

Only some of the instruments used during the dental visit need to be sterilized. For instance, the dental burs (the actual parts that contact teeth in drilling and polishing) are either sterilized or discarded between patients. All dental offices have extra sets of instruments to allow for proper sterilization time. To ensure that the instruments are appropriately sterilized, they are first soaked in a chemical cleaning solution and then either hand scrubbed or cleaned with an ultrasonic device, which removes debris by means of vibration.

Generally, instruments that do not penetrate oral tissue or bone need only be disinfected, not sterilized. This includes plastic film holders used to take radiographs (x-rays) and metal or plastic impression trays.

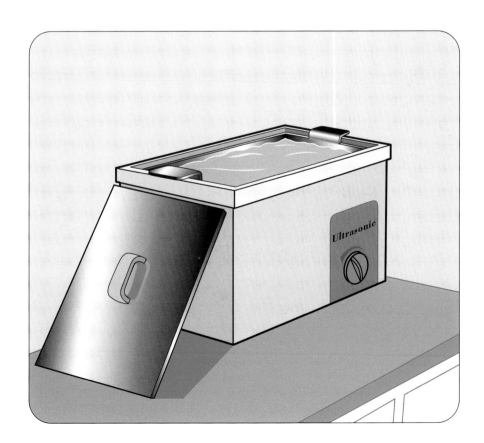

Is There a Way to Be Sure That Sterilization Has Worked?

Because sterilization is so important to infection control, the dental team regularly monitors or tests all sterilization equipment.

Chemical monitoring is accomplished with the use of a special ink. A strip of heat-sensitive ink is included in the package with the instruments during the sterilization process. The ink changes color when the required temperature has been reached. This ink change then signals to the dental team that packaged instruments have been exposed to the proper temperature.

Biological spore testing is done by testing the sterilization process on harmless live bacteria, which are contained in sealed vials. Biological spore monitoring is considered a more reliable method of measuring the effectiveness of sterilization. It is accomplished by exposing difficult-to-destroy bacteria to the normal sterilization process and verifying that these bacteria have in fact been destroyed. If sterilization was not successful, the instruments are *not* used on patients and the sterilizer is repaired or replaced.

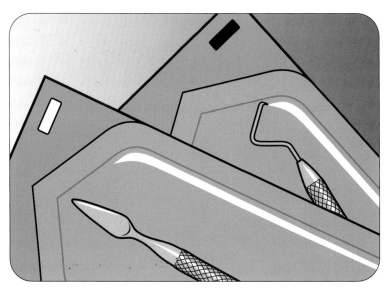

While biological monitoring is the key way to ensure that only sterilized instruments are used in treatment, chemical monitoring is also used. On these sterilization packets are heat-sensitive ink strips. When instruments have undergone sterilization, the strips change color, indicating to the dental team that the instruments are safe to use.

Can Dental Handpieces Transmit Infection?

Some reports in the media have suggested that dental handpieces (the instrument holding the dental drill) could possibly transmit HIV. These reports suggested that the debris from one patient's mouth could become lodged inside a dental handpiece and then be expelled during the treatment of another patient. No transmission of any pathogen, however, has ever been documented by this route. Furthermore, dental offices sterilize their handpieces between patients, killing all potential disease-causing organisms, including the AIDS virus.

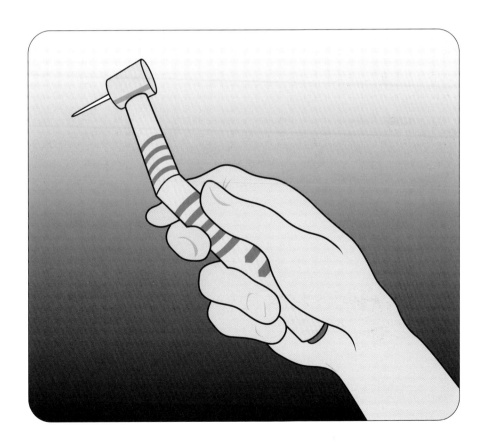

Where Does the Infectious Waste Go?

Disposal of all infectious waste generated in dental offices is governed by federal, state, and local laws and regulations. Special containers, called biohazard containers, are used to store the waste before licensed haulers remove it from the dental office. Such waste is delivered to government-approved processing sites, where it is decontaminated and destroyed. These processing sites are strictly regulated by the federal government and the Environmental Protection Agency.

Burs and other sharp disposable materials that may be used in the course of dental procedures have special containers for disposal. These "sharps" are placed in designated containers that are puncture resistant, leakproof, and specially labeled. Like other infectious waste, their disposal is governed by various regulations.

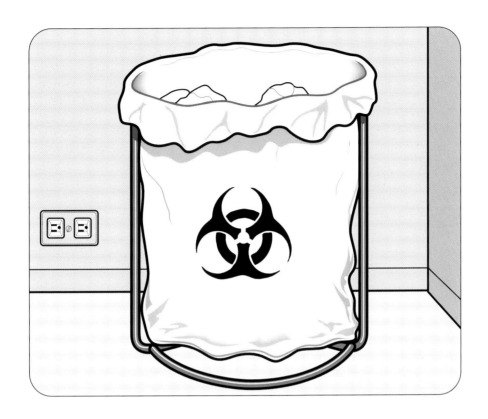

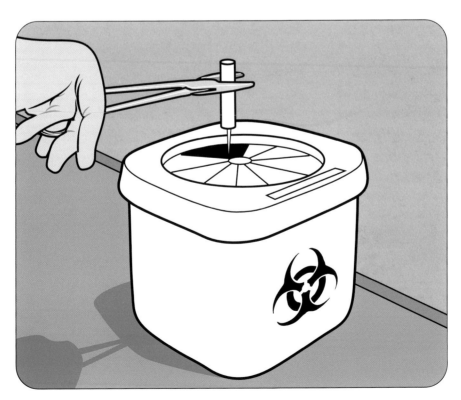

Biohazard container (top). For safety, used needles and other sharp objects are disposed in a designated container called a sharps disposal *(above).*

What About AIDS ?

Transmission of HIV occurs through contact with blood, intimate sexual contact, and from HIV-infected mothers to their newborns. Casual contact has never been known to transmit HIV. **HIV cannot be transmitted by tears, urine, sweat, dental aerosol, or insect bites.** Furthermore, HIV is a very fragile virus—it is easily killed by disinfectants regularly used in dental offices.

Recent studies have suggested that saliva contains components that render HIV harmless. In fact, these factors that inhibit HIV are being widely studied and one day may be used to treat HIV disease.

HIV has not been shown to be transmitted even when blood is present in saliva. Thus, being a patient in a dental office that treats HIV-infected patients does not pose any risk. However, even if there were a chance that HIV could be transmitted in a dental office, adherence to "universal precautions" would virtually eliminate such an occurrence. Furthermore, it is probably safe to presume that dental offices that knowingly treat HIV-infected patients will have the best infection control available!

The Controversy

Since the initial reports of HIV-infected patients in the early 1980s, the possible transmission of HIV in health-care settings has been debated both among health-care providers and in the lay press. Concern heightened in 1990, when CDC, the federal watchdog agency for public health policy, reported a possible transmission of HIV from a dentist with AIDS to one of his patients. Since that time, five additional patients have come forward claiming to have been infected by the same dentist.

Numerous investigations have tried to explain if and how such a transmission might have occurred, but none have succeeded in doing so. Furthermore, even today, this case remains a puzzle, as no mode of transmission has been detected and no other cases have been found where HIV-infected health-care providers have been implicated in the transmission of HIV to patients. In fact, the opposite seems to be true. Studies of over 22,000 patients treated by 51 HIV-infected health-care providers, 29 of them dentists and dental students, could not document a *single case* of HIV transmission from an infected health-care provider to a patient.

Because HIV is so fragile, and because all equipment and surfaces that may have been contaminated are cleaned and disinfected between each and every patient, it's not surprising that HIV transmission between patients has never been documented in a dental office.

Is It Safe to Go to the Dental Office?

Yes! You now know that all dental equipment is replaced, disinfected, or sterilized between patients. In some cases, additional protective barriers are used to facilitate cleaning. You may notice plastic or latex wraps or aluminum foil on the light handles or covering the chair controls in the dental office. All of these measures are ways of ensuring your safety in the dental setting.

Dental offices that use appropriate infection-control techniques and routinely practice "universal precautions" for all dental procedures are safe. The members of the dental team care very much about your safety and follow every known recommendation to prevent the transmission of disease in the dental setting.

Because of the increasing sophistication of infection-control measures, your dental office has never been safer.

What Your Dentist Does
to Keep the Dental Office Safe

- Employs "universal precautions" for all patients
- Uses and reviews the health history form of all patients
- Immunizes herself/himself and all staff against hepatitis B
- Follows OSHA/ADA/CDC recommendations and guidelines
- Regularly attends infection-control update courses and integrates new practices into the dental office
- Uses protective barriers such as glasses, gloves, masks, and gowns
- Disinfects patient treatment areas before each patient
- Sterilizes the dental instruments and handpieces
- Monitors disinfection and sterilization solutions for efficacy
- Monitors sterilizers for efficacy
- Disposes of infectious waste according to federal, state, and local laws

About the Authors

Michael Glick, DMD, is Associate Professor of Oral Medicine and Director of the Infectious Disease Program at the University of Pennsylvania School of Dental Medicine. He is the recipient of numerous awards for his educational and research efforts, and he serves on national and international committees on HIV and other blood-borne infectious diseases. In 1995 he was appointed to the ADA Council on Scientific Affairs. Dr. Glick is the author of *Dental Management of Patients with HIV*.

Brian C. Muzyka, DMD, is Assistant Professor at Louisiana State University School of Dentistry, Department of Oral Medicine, and Louisiana State University Medical Center, New Orleans, Louisiana. He received his post-doctoral specialty training in oral medicine at the University of Pennsylvania School of Dental Medicine and a clinical fellowship at the University of Pennsylvania Medical Center. Dr. Muzyka has written extensively on oral medicine.